HOW TO ACQUIRE SUPER-STRENGTH

BY
OTTO ARCO

Official title-holder: "The World's Strongest Man"

Originally Published in 1932

PUBLISHED BY O'Faolain Patriot LLC,
Copyright 2012

info@PhysicalCultureBooks.com

Published in the United States of America

ISBN-13: 978-1477633106

ISBN-10: 1477633103

To Order More Copies Visit: Physical Culture
Books.com

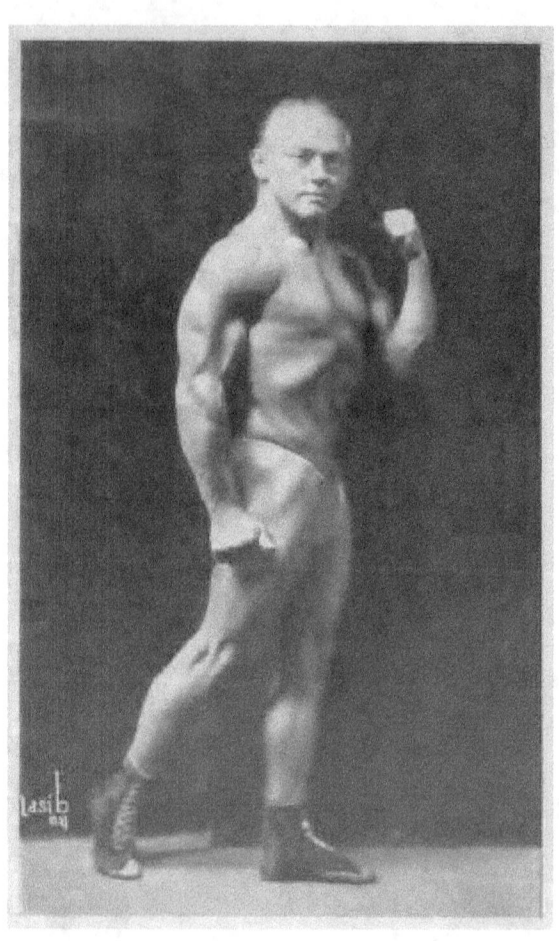

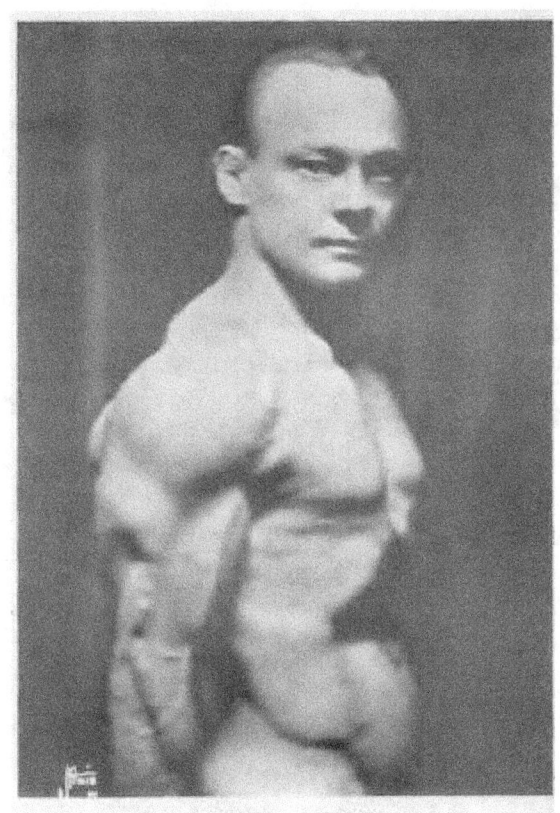

OTTO ARCO
Winner of the Official, International Title
"The World's Best Developed Man"

AN APPRECIATION BY HIS FRIEND
STANISLAUS ZBYSZKO.

Otto Arco is the marvel of physical culture experts, the idol of countless physical culture fans all over the world. He has one of the most magnificent builds that any man has ever developed. Arco is master of that difficult art of muscle-control, perfect co-ordination which is the secret of all great feats of strength. For thirty years Arco has demonstrated his spectacular strength, appearing in leading world's theatres. Otto Arco is recognized everywhere not only as a perfect physical specimen himself, but as the foremost exponent of physical culture. I have met many who said that a few words from Otto Arco have helped them more than years of study and exercise under other physical culture instructors.

(signed) STANISLAUS ZBYSZKO.

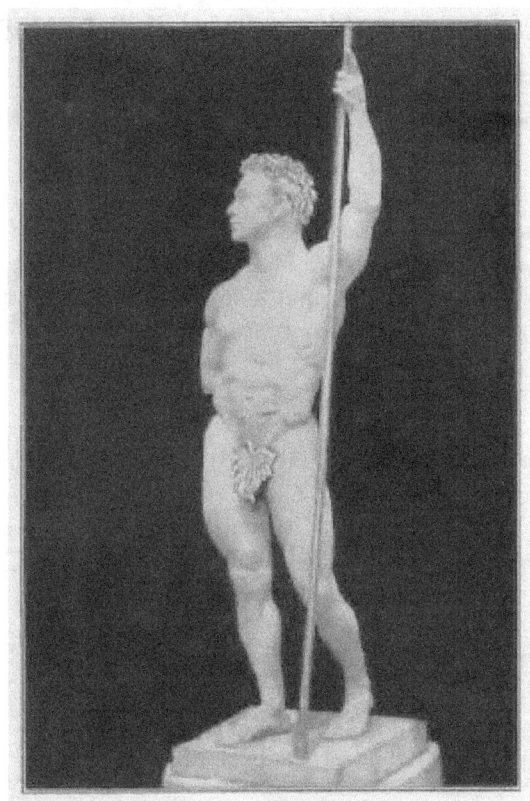

A classical pose showing the proportions and muscular development of my body.

A WORD FROM ALAN CALVERT, ONE OF THE WORLD'S GREATEST AUTHORITIES ON PHYSICAL CULTURE.

To whom it may concern.

I am informed that Otto Arco is going to give Instructions in Physical Culture. I would congratulate any one that had the good fortune to secure the services of Arco as an instructor.

Arco is unquestionably one of the best developed men in the history of athletics—has had vast experience, and his knowledge of exercise and proper body building methods is almost unlimited. I admire him as an athlete and have always been impressed with his ability to teach; above all, I respect his reliability and high personal character.

I do no personal teaching myself, but if a man or boy told me that individual instruction was what he wanted, I would recommend Arco as being away ahead of any other instructor in his line of work.

(Signed) ALAN CALVERT.

HOW TO ACQUIRE SUPER-STRENGTH

BY OTTO ARCO.

NO TWO MEN are made alike. That is one of the remarkable truths of life. You are different from anybody else in build, chemical make-up, constitution, temperament and physical condition.

Obviously, these individual factors should be taken into consideration in any program of physical-training that you undertake. You know, for example, that everybody cannot eat the same foods. "What's one man's meat is another man's poison." Some things may be good for you that are injurious to others. And vice versa, a diet that may be beneficial to another person may not agree with your system.

The same thing applies to exercise. A program of training that builds up another man and develops his strength may tend to weaken you, rather than strengthen you.

It is not only a question of the amount of exercise; it has to do with the kind of exercise as well. In like manner, your entire program of training should be based upon your individual needs and requirements.

How Wrong Methods Can Hurt You

I cannot impress this fact upon you too strongly. I have seen so many promising fellows retarded by wrong training methods. In some cases the heart has been over-strained, in others an excessive loss of weight has resulted with a lowering of resistance and vitality; many men have become what they call "muscle-bound", so that they can never acquire any real strength.

Scarcely a day passes but what men write to me and ask why they have not gotten the expected benefits from exercise. Some of them have tried practically every system under the sun. Many have exercised for years without being any better off than when they started.

A Typical Example

Just recently a young chap paid me a visit. He had a very promising build and development, but he was in pitiful condition. It seems that he was ambitious to become an athletic instructor, and had gone to a well-known professional instructor of strong men for advice. For a substantial sum of money this man had laid out a program of training for him. The result was that inside of a week the enthusiastic pupil had torn the tendons of his shoulder and legs so that he was scarcely able to move. Of course these would heal in time, although they might always remain as "weak points" that would have to be humored in any athletic activities. I dread to think what might have happened if this man had continued with the training program laid out for him, for it was beyond his physical capacity at the time. It was not only that it was too strenuous for his strength; it was not adapted to his physical make-up. He was a tall, rangy man and required a special type of exercise adapted to his build.

Muscles Cannot be Turned Out by a Factory

I am not criticising this particular instructor. He simply recommended a routine that he had found satisfactory in his own case, and unfortunately that is the basis of most of the courses of physical culture that are offered. In fact, some of these courses are printed by the thousands. They are sold without discrimination to the weak and the strong, the young and the old alike. Men who enroll for these standardized courses may consider themselves fortunate if they derive no harm from them. And as for the benefits expected, I am constantly receiving letters from men who have followed such courses blindly and cannot understand why they have obtained no results.

Yet the reason is obvious. What would you think of a physician who prescribed for you without ever seeing you, without giving any study to your particular condition? Wouldn't you be afraid to take the medicine he sent you? You should be just as careful about selecting your program of physical culture. Don't make the mistake of thinking that any exercise is good for you. Exercise can hurt you just as it can help you. In many instances too much exercise, no matter how good or seemingly effective, will do greater harm than none at all. By following some standardized course of instructions or illustrated chart many unknowingly overdo and sometimes seriously injure themselves.

My Method is Different

I think I may say without boasting, that I KNOW physical culture. It has been my life study and profession. The fact that I built up my own body to the perfection that won for me the official, international title of the "World's Best Developed Man", and that I developed my strength to the extent of breaking worlds records in official contests, should be convincing evidence that my methods work.

But the mere fact that a man is strong himself does not necessarily qualify him to instruct others. Even more important than my own record as a strong man from your standpoint is the fact that I have made a lifelong study of physical culture methods. I have travelled all over the world, I have trained with the world's greatest athletes and compared notes with them, including such great, stars as Arthur Saxon, George Hackenschmidt, Maxick, Steinbach, Pandour Brothers, Zbyszko, Klein,

Swoboda, Thomas Inch, Sandow, Apollon, Deriaz Brothers and many others. I have been an active member of the athletic clubs of Europe, France, Germany, Austria, Russia, Poland and America. I know the methods used by the leading strong men here and abroad. I know which methods have proven most effective —and above everything else, I know that every man's training must be designed to fit his particular condition and needs. With the right training there is no reason why any man cannot develop great strength and build up his body progressively to ideal proportions.

Throughout my long experience I have seen overwhelming proof of what the right training methods will do for a man. For nearly 30 years I travelled all over the world, playing the leading theatres as a headline attraction. Thousands of physical culturists visited me back stage. Famous strong men and athletes came to my dressing room to talk over training methods and to ask my advice. I analyzed their methods, noted the best points and in this way accumulated a vast fund of knowledge covering every conceivable phase of physical culture.

Many aspiring young fellows also came to me for advice and it was always a great pleasure to help these ambitious chaps along the road to their goal. It was most gratifying, too, to note the results of my advice and some of the leading strong men of today attribute their success to the friendly coaching I gave them "back stage".

There is, for example, Walter Podolak, who is today acclaimed the Strongest Man in America, and who holds the world's amateur record for a dead lift of 654 pounds. Walter first called on me at a theatre in Syracuse, when he was a lad 15 years old. He told me of his ambitions to develop himself and I started him off on a program of instruction. His progress was amazing and if you will look at the photo of Walter Podolak, shown elsewhere in this book, you will understand my pride in having been of some service in helping to develop so fine a specimen of manhood.

Another young chap who came to see me while he was still in his teens was Tommy Faber. He was a slightly built boy, but well proportioned and he had a consuming ambition to become a professional strong man. I gave him the instruction he needed and he went to work. As a result he developed one of the finest physiques I have ever seen. Later I gave him a place in my "strong man" act where his magnificent build and his great strength won him wide recognition.

I could cite many other instances of men whom I have helped to achieve distinction in physical culture. I do not say this boastfully, I merely want to point out the results that are secured by following the right methods. Above all, let me emphasize once more the all-important fact that each man's training must be based on his individual condition and planned to meet his particular needs.

In addition to the thousands of personal visits I have received from men anxious to learn my "secrets" of developing great muscular power, I have had letters from many Physical Culture Instructors and Physicians of prominence all over the world seeking my advice and guidance. In each case I made a careful study and analysis of each individual before advising him what to do, and the many grateful letters I have received in return are a glowing testimonial to the success of my instructions.

It was as a result of this world-wide demand for my personal help that I set about to devise a plan whereby 1 could make my instruction available to all who desired it. I formulated my Questionnaire, or personal analysis blank, so that I might have all the necessary information about each individual on which to base his instruction. From a study of this, 1 am able to write each man personally, telling him just what to do to solve his particular problems, to achieve his particular ends and to reach his highest development in health, strength and muscles.

Not an Ordinary "Correspondence Course"

Now, while I give this personal instruction by correspondence, I do not want you to think of it as an ordinary "correspondence course". I do NOT print up my lessons in advance. I do not give you a standardized set of instructions to all who enroll with me. To the best of my knowledge, I am the only physical culture instructor who writes each man personally and gives him really personal instruction designed exclusively for him.

My instruction is, so to speak, "custom built" to your own specifications. It applies to you only because it is made to your individual measure. That, in my opinion, is the only way that physical culture instruction should be given, and while I could perhaps make a great deal more money by turning out standardized lessons in wholesale quantities, my own conscience would not allow me to do so. I know that such instruction not only would not do you any substantial good, but it might actually harm you.

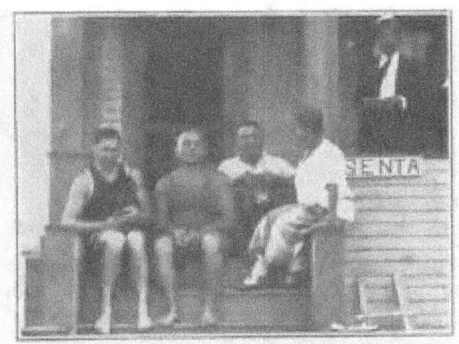

Jack Dempsey, Zbyszko, myself and Mrs. Zbyszko at the Zbyszko cottage in Maine. Dempsey spent quite a fine time with us while on a hunting and fishing trip through Maine.

The Short-Cut to Health, Strength, Muscles

My instruction does get results. It gets them first, because it is planned to lit your individual needs— and secondly, because it employs the very best of all physical culture methods. It is the "cream" of the accumulated knowledge not only of myself, but of all the world's leading athletes and strong men. This expert knowledge is absolutely priceless to any man who wants to reach the highest point in strength and physical development.

Enormous progress has been made in physical culture training as in everything else. If you are sticking to the old way; trying to pump up your muscles to any desired shape with all sorts of old-fashioned, tedious movements, you are just one of the many thousands who are working for little or no results.

My method is in no way related to the antiquated and obsolete systems so much in use. It does not strain, tax or wear you out. It is simple and pleasant, logical and natural. It eliminates all the old-fashioned and unnecessary routine and gets results with the minimum expenditure of time, money and muscular energy.

How I Plan Your Training Program

After analyzing your physical possibilities and deficiencies I will prescribe the method of exercise best suited to your condition. I have a special way, the result of thirty-five years of actual experience, of explaining and simplifying everything I want to tell you. The exercises I prescribe are of an entirely different sort. You will realize their effectiveness the minute you begin using them. And you will enjoy your exercising periods instead of dreading them as many still do.

My system also includes a program of proper diet, posture, breathing, self-control, the general care of your body and many other important things pertaining to your condition. Nothing is overlooked that will be of help to you.

If I cannot help you, I doubt if anyone can. That is the way I feel and I can prove it. Not by empty words but by the many unsolicited testimonials from pupils. A large proportion of these are from men who have tried other methods and acknowledge that my method is the only one that has brought them the desired result of a perfect, strong and healthy body.

In all sincerity, I can say to you that if you really want to develop your body and increase your strength, I can show you how to do it in the shortest possible time and with the least effort. You will get results in a fraction of the usual time—and you will get results that you could never achieve with other systems.

As to the Use of Weights

I regard weights as a natural means of securing resistance with exercises, and if your condition warrants and you have weights at home, I may recommend the use of them. If I do, it will be in a way you will enjoy rather than dread, as some do. So if you are one of those who dislikes the idea of using weights, rest assured that I will not try to force the use of them upon you.

However, if you are interested in weight-lifting, I will positively increase your lifting capacity. By systematic preparatory exercises, proved by the best European lifters, I will accomplish for you in a short time results which you have perhaps been striving for years to obtain. It is all in "knowing how", as every experienced weight-lifter will realize. We have many strong boys here in America, but they are no match for their European competitors, simply because they do not know the right way. This was evident during the last Olympic contests when our boys made such a poor showing. As I watched these boys in training, I realized that they would never measure up, because they were not getting the proper instruction.

And so, whatever may be your particular interest or ambition in physical culture, I know that the proper kind of instruction will make a tremendous difference in the results you obtain, and the ease and speed with which you obtain them.

A Word to the Young Man

You are at the critical stage in your training. Your whole future success in physical culture depends upon getting the right start. Wrong exercise, wrong training can do harm that can never be undone. Your body is still in the formative stage, your muscles are not yet fully developed. Be careful! Make sure that you are on the right track, that you have proper guidance before you go ahead with any program of exercise.

I have seen scores of young men incapacitated so that they will never be able to realize their finest development and achieve great strength simply because they went ahead blindly with exercise unsuited to their condition and special needs. Many young men knot up their muscles through over-taxing them so that they can never regain the flexibility and elasticity that are vital to strength.

Your training should above all be geared to your present development and physical condition. Only in this way can your body be built up step by step to its highest perfection. Now more than at any time, you need the personal guidance of an expert, who will study you carefully and advise you as to what to do and what not to do.

Believe me, I am very deeply in earnest when I say this to you—so earnest, in fact, that even if you do not enroll with me for my instruction,

I wish you would at least fill out my questionnaire and return it to me for my examination. Rather than see you go wrong, I will be glad to advise you as to the type of training you should follow, entirely free of charge.

A Word to You Older Men

Not a few of the men who write to me arc getting along in years and beginning to feel that they are slipping. They want to know if I can help them to retain their youth, their vitality and physical fitness. If there is anything like the "Fountain of Youth", 1 believe I have the nearest thing to it. I am a man of fifty with the body of a youngster. It is my own system of exercising that is responsible for my condition, the same system that you will receive when you subscribe for my personal instructions.

But whatever your age or present condition, I KNOW, out of my years of experience, that my system of personal instruction will literally make a new man out of you. Do you want muscles? I will cover your body with layers of them, shapely, powerful muscles packed with genuine strength. Do you want health? I will charge your body with the vibrant joy of living, I will tone and strengthen your internal organs; I will put you in the pink of condition so that you will eat well, sleep well, and feel well. Have you some special problem that you want to take up with me? My friendly counsel and advice are at your service.

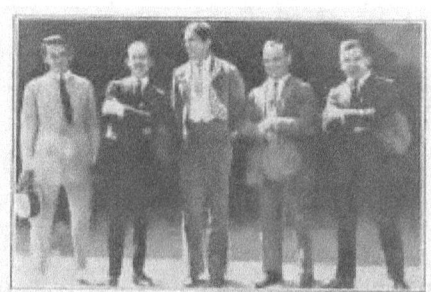

Here you see me with some of the Hollywood celebrities. L. to R.: Richard Talmadge, his brother, Douglas Fairbanks, myself, and my brother. Doug and I did some fine hand-to-hand balancing stunts just before this picture was taken. What a pity I could not get a snapshot of this.

ONE OF MY FAMOUS PUPILS

WALTER PODOLAK, WORLD'S STRONGEST MAN

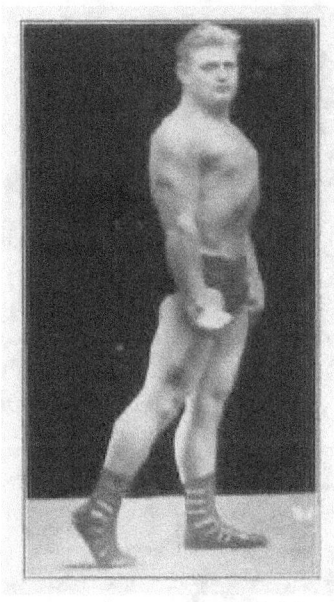

Who does not know Walter Podolak, of Syracuse, N. Y., one of the greatest strong men of our time, who is credited by such authorities as Mark Berry, with being the strongest man in the world. Walter holds the amateur world's record in the dead weight lift with a lift of 454½ lbs. He lifted more than Goerner unofficially and he would easily have won first place in the last Olympic meet had he not turned professional just a few months before. However, Walter has little cause for regret as he is very successful and earns a handsome income.

Walter received my first instructions at fifteen, followed them faithfully and WON.

SOME OF MY PUPILS

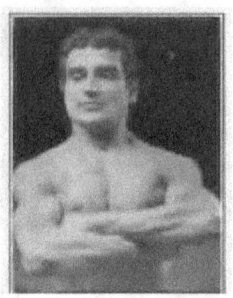

Michael Sulvane of Worcester, Mass. A real anatomic wonder, he could easily serve as a muscle chart, so finely defined are all of the different muscle groups. A conscientious follower of the physical culture life, Michael has devoted himself enthusiastically to my instructions, with wonderful results.

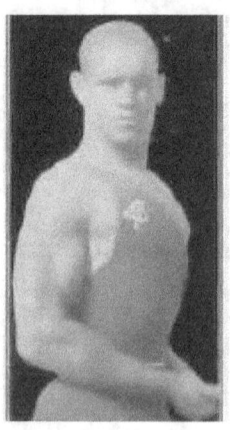

Albert Hunte of Bridgetown, Barbadoes, B. W. I.
one of the strongest boys of the B. W. I. In part he
writes: "I'm glad I enrolled with you. Have made
wonderful progress and would recommend you to
anyone who wishes a super-physique. Your weight-
balancing instructions are great and nothing could
replace them. Nothing like it on the market."

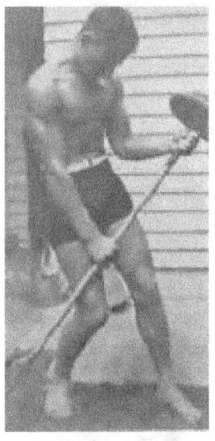

W. Hyde of Napier, N. Z. says that after following
my program for three months, he has put on 10 lbs
of solid muscle and increased his two-arm lifts by
42 lbs.

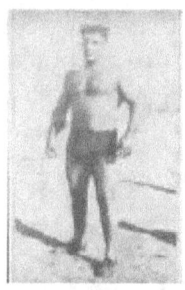

Harry Ekizian, former wrestling champion of U. S.
Navy. One of the most enthusiastic followers of
My System. He says that since he started My Way
he increased his bodily strength almost twofold.
Although fairly light for a professional wrestler he
tosses some of the big fellows around as if they
were lightweights, he has a good contract with the
movies now and enjoys a great deal of success.

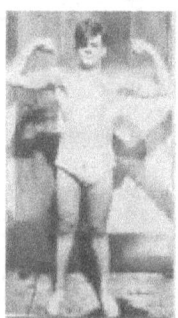

Walter Manning, of Phila. Pa. has some American
amateur weight lifting records to his credit since he
started to train My Way. Look at his physique. This
snapshot scarcely does him justice, for Walter has a

really superb physique, with powerfully developed muscles whose measurements would be a source of pride to any man.

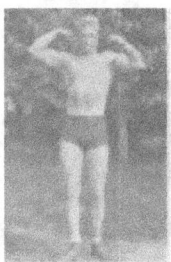

Alfred Hedlund of Oakland, Cal. has also the makings of a future professional wrestling champion. A six-footer, young, energetic and look at those proportions. Alfred has the build of an Apollo—and the strength of a Hercules. I prophesize great things for him.

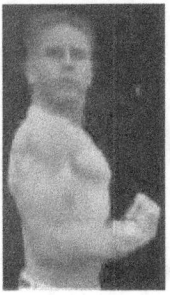

John Patrick Jesse of Los Angeles, Cal. reports that he has gained 12 lbs. of muscle in a little more than

one month after changing to the training program
which I outlined for him.

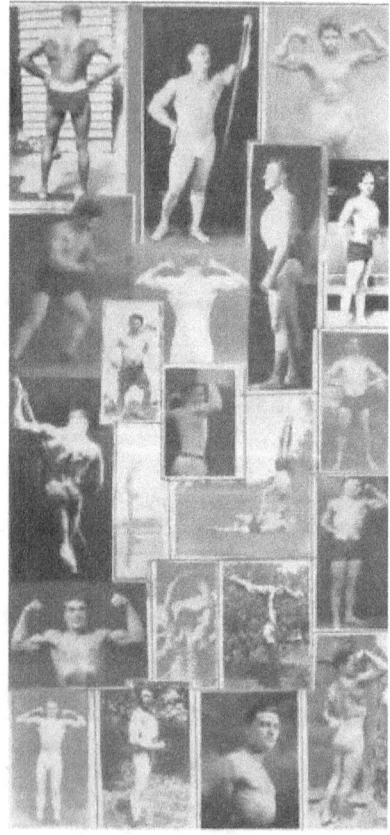

Here are some of my pupils—unretouched
photographs voluntarily sent to me to show the
progress being made under my instruction. Every

one of these men is enthusiastic about my methods. They enjoy training my way— and they are getting results. Over and over again pupils write to me to say that a few weeks of training under my direction have done more for them than years of laborious, tedious exercising under old-fashioned systems.

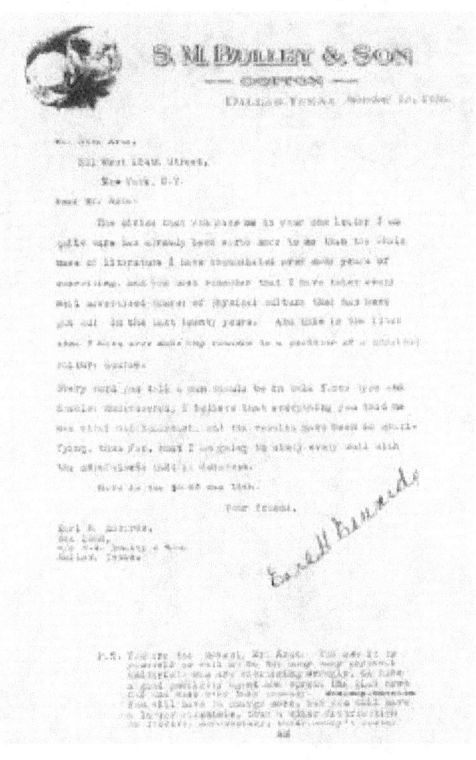

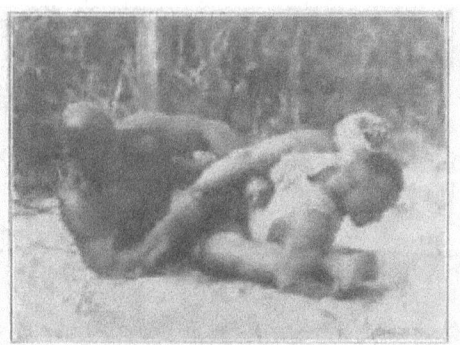

Here you see me and Stanislaus Zbyszko engaging in a friendly wrestling bout on the Old Orchard Beach.

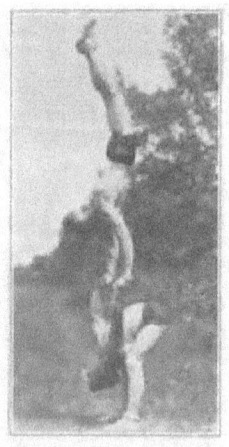

VICTOR OLSON Gold Medal Winner and Handbalancing Artist says: "By your valuable instructions I have improved my act one hundred per cent and am qualified to play any engage- now. You are the greatest teacher of them all."

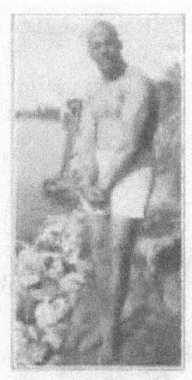

MAH EL BASSIUNI Physical Director of H. M. King of Egypt's Army is one of my most distinguished pupils. He is the one who has trained and coached E. S. M. Noseir the present Amateur Heavyweight Champion of the World. He says, in part: "My desire is to be like you till I die."

<u>TESTIMONIALS (CONTINUED)</u>

Another Example of What My Instruction Accomplishes.

Dear Mr. Arco:

I have followed everything you wrote me in your letter and must say that I feel 75% better. Your one letter has helped me more than the five months of needless exercising and waste of time and money. The diet you prescribed for me has helped me very much. I have no more pains in the stomach and no headaches.

JOSEPH ZAWISTOWSKI,

Bayonne, N. J.

Some Professional Opinions

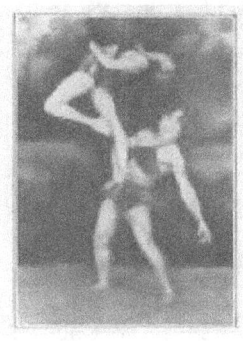

Robert Ra Nous, one of America's greatest athletes and foremost Adagio dancers, says: "When it comes to practical advice on Physical Training, I know of no one that can give it better than Arco. I have benefitted immensely by his wonderful and unexcelled advice."

Extracts from an article in "Body Molding" Magazine.

"I knew of Otto Arco before he left Europe as one of the best developed men of all times and one of the strongest of his size. He was world-famous before he ever came to America. Arco, to my mind, is the gnat exception among professional 'strong men.' He is one of the very few of that class who is interested in bodily culture for its own sake. He has helped hundred of men with his advice and counsel; did it all from a spirit of helpfulness."

Here is what LILLIAN LEITZEL, World's Greatest Woman Gymnast and Athlete, Star Attraction, Ringling Bros., Barnuni & Bailey Circus, thinks of me:

Dear Friend Arco:

I was pleased to hear that you finally started in the teaching of Physical Culture.

Knowing you for so long, and also your enthusiasm and devotion to Physical Culture, I don't doubt but that you will do a world of good to anyone who becomes your pupil.

Assuring you of my sincere wishes for your great success, I remain with my best personal regards,

(Signed) LILLIAN LEITZEL.

RICHARD TALMADGE also thinks well of me:

Dear Arco:

I know that with your knowledge on the subject of Physical Development you will work wonders with anyone who comes under your guidance and direction. I am sure you are bound to be a huge success in the Physical Culture field.

Sincerely,

(Signed) RICHARD TALMADGE,

Universal City, California.

WII.LIAM J. HERRMANN, Philadelphia's great Physical Culture teacher, writes:

Fortunate, indeed, will be those that will consult you, and astonishing results will be shown. It will be my pleasure to recommend you to all interested in building up and perfecting their bodies.

(Signed) WM. J. HERRMANN.

SIGMUND KLEIN, America's strongest and best developed specimen of manhood says:

"I would recommend Otto Arco to any individual without the least hesitation as an undisputed authority on all matters concerning strength and development."

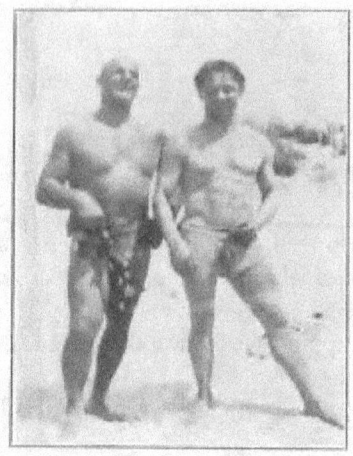

An informal snapshot of Zbyszko and myself on the beach at Old Orchard, Me. I have spent many happy times with my famous friend at his summer cottage, where we were visited by many of the world's leading athletes.

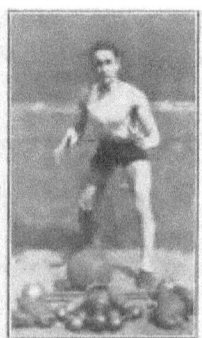 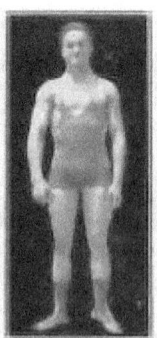

(At left) Charles Scharffer, of Williamsburg, N. Y. as he was at the age of 16 and, on right, as he looked one year later, after he started to follow my system and advice. One of the finest examples of what the right way of training can do for anybody.

TESTIMONIALS (CONTINUED)

I am enclosing here the balance I owe because you say that when I obtain results I can pay. Believe me I did obtain results so I owe this to you.

G. THIBAUDEAU, Quebec, P. Q.

Received your Balancing outfit a few weeks ago and sure think it's a wonderful thing to own. One thing that is so good is that it serves as an all around developer.

JOE ORTOLANI, Rochester, N. Y.

I am delighted with the personal and individual way you have of instructing. Your system and opinions are certainly entirely different from any of well known Physical Instructors. Logical, sound and much more pleasant and interesting than any system I have ever followed before. Your instructions have certainly given me an entirely new slant on the subject of P. C. and inspired me with a new zest in the whole thing.

CECIL C. HYNDMAN, Ottawa, Ont.

I must say that your instructions are the finest ever and although I have not exercised as regularly as I would like to, the results are splendid. I like the simplicity of the exercises. No bother loading and unloading plates which before always grew monotonous. In following your instructions I get a wonderful workout and always end up feeling fine.

CLYDE S. REED.

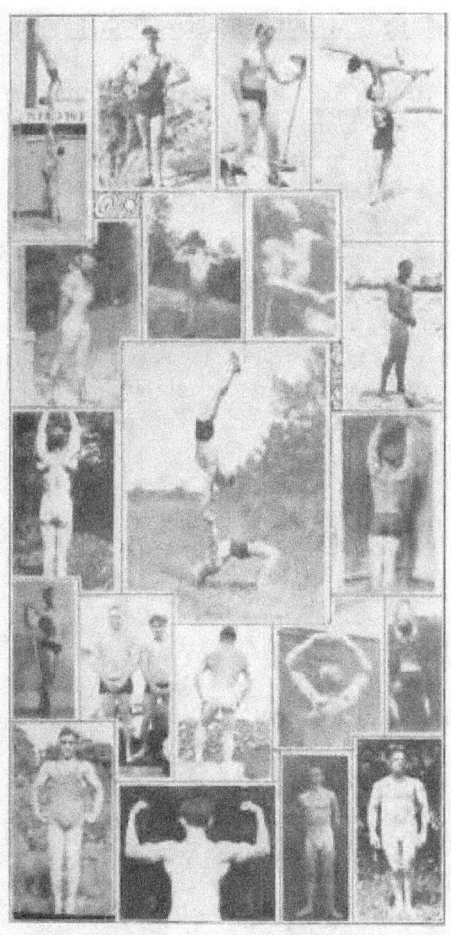

Another page of my pupils, all of them great boosters of my methods. Beginner or professional strong man, I give each man just the instruction he needs to accomplish the maximum results in the shortest possible time. The glowing tributes of my pupils speak volumes for the effectiveness of my training. The remarkable results obtained only go to show what expert, individual instruction can do for any man.

Testimonials (continued)

My Trapezius has developed to a high extent through your course since I last wrote you and my pectorals are tremendously big with that rounded-out effect on the upper part.

JOHN P. JESSE, Los Angeles, Calif.

I was certainly delighted with my progress under your direction; you should have seen what I looked like about 14 months ago. I only weighed 107 lbs. I certainly am glad I picked your course from the 20 or so that I have inquired about.

HENRY D. STUART, Chilliwack, B. C., Canada.

Thought I would drop you a few lines and let you know how I have gotten along with your exceedingly good course.

For the short time I have followed your instructions I can honestly say that I have never seen such exercises as those which you teach with a bar bell that give such a large amount of stamina and endurance to a fellow.

After I work out as per your instructions I have so much pep and vigor that I feel as though I could box ten rounds without any let-down.

HOWARD J. GRIFFIN.

No one could help but be benefitted by your advice and I feel that I am getting "straight dope" from you.

WILLIAM R. RICHARDSON.

I have received your course and I am very happy to have subscribed to same. It certainly looks like the very thing I have been in quest of for the last eight years and I sincerely hope that my quest for strength and development ends right here with your course. You are absolutely correct when you state that bar bell repetition exercises burns one's energy up, because when I finished my bar bell exercises I felt completely fagged out, my hands trembled and felt like never wanting to exercise again. I certainly felt terrible, no pep, etc. Your course is just the opposite, I feel fine when I am through and full of pep.

GEORGE A. NAMI.

"I wish to thank you a thousand times for the wonderful results I have thus far received from your great course and I wish to say that the small amount which you ask for your course is but a trifle compared to the good results received from same. Yes, your course is worth many times more than you ask for it."

"Mr. Arco, I received the three photos of you O. K. I am very glad indeed to have them. They showed the results of your methods of training to a wonderful degree."

"Have improved wonderfully all around since started to follow your advice."

"Am glad I wrote you, I am well repaid."

"I am forced to write and tell you how much better I am since you told me of my mistakes."

"Have gained 6 lbs. since started your instructions, and it is all muscle, too."

"The way you explain everything is wonderful and I can see now my mistakes plainly."

"I thought there was nothing new under the sun to know about Physical Training until I read your letter with instructions."

"Your weight balancing outfit is about the best idea of modern exercising I have tested in a long time."

-x-x-x-

I have hundreds of letters, from many friends, who thank me for the splendid results that they achieved through my advice. If you seriously wish to improve your present condition, join our crowd!

PHOTOGRAPHS OF MYSELF

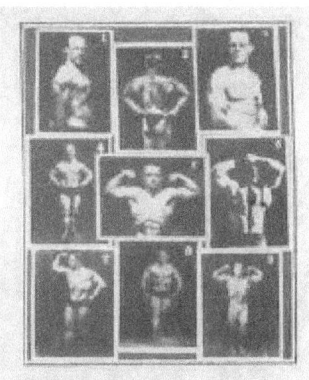

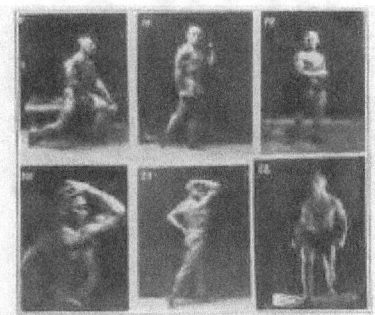

So many admirers of physical development have written to me for photographs of myself that I have had 15 different poses made up as shown here. These are all original photographs, size 8x10, and I will be glad to supply any of them for 50c a piece or 5 for $2.00—Order by number. Enlargements may be had at proportionate prices.

AUTOGRAPHED IF DESIRED.

Any two photos included free of charge if you enroll for my instruction. State which two you desire with your enrollment.

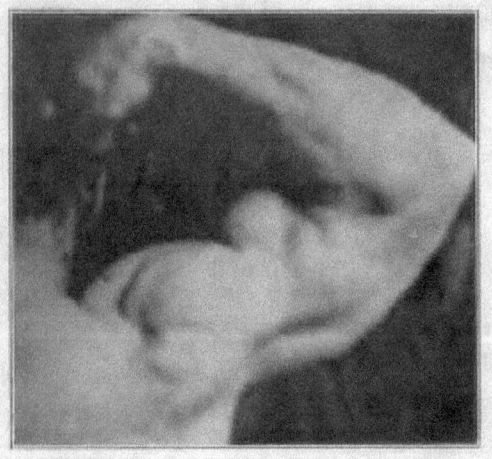

Do you want an arm like this? This is an unretouched photo of my own arm as it appeared in Strength Magazine.

A FINAL WORD.

I have told you how I can help you to realize your fullest possibilities for health and strength in the shortest possible time, through my exclusive method of individual instruction; I have given you the statements of foremost physical culture authorities as to my qualifications and knowledge; I have shown you the testimony of some of my pupils who have actually proved my way to health and strength.

Still, I realize that it is difficult to make you believe my claims, for after all, everybody can make the same claims. Since I started giving individual instruction by mail, most of the other instructors have added the words "personal instruction" to their promises, but would you call lessons that are printed by the thousands "personal" or "individual"?

The instruction you get from me is prepared for you alone and for nobody else. That, in my opinion, is the only kind of instruction that can be truthfully called personal and individual and the only effective method to get lasting results for your effort in less time and with the least waste of energy' and money.

When you enroll for my instruction it is like consulting a specialist. You get advice to meet your own special requirements. Yet my fee is actually less than is commonly charged by ordinary, standardized courses that are nothing more nor less than so many printed pages. I am a physical culture enthusiast myself—I am glad to make my experience and advice available to others. I have tried to bring it within reach of all. I hope that I may have the pleasure of extending to you my sincere personal interest and wholehearted co-operation.

OTTO ARCO